Essential oils. The ethereal molecules of the plants

Anti-inflammatory and antimicrobial essential oils and how they work

Crystal Leeper

Table of contents

Ancient knowledge of essential oils 7

How are essential oils absorbed by our bodies? 10

The influence of essential oils on our state of being 12

The beneficial properties of essential oils 16

Anti-inflammatory and antibacterial recipes 16

Plant biology 19

Essential oils compounds 22

Extraction 25

A bottle of divine potion on the supermarket shelf 27

The great wonders of nature have always found a way to infiltrate in our consciousness and affect great revelations about ourselves and about our subtle interactions with the world around. Our favorite path is a methodological one by which ration guides us into studying, analyzing, experimenting, demonstrating and postulating. This scientific approach hasn't yet succeeded in explaining the miraculously healing effect of a simple walk through a field of blossomed chamomile, yarrow, marjoram. The benefits have been stated and proved, but such a beautiful manner to administer a medicine, as to literally inhale the therapeutic contents of a plant, is still something to be understood by employing intuition. And in this line of thought, grasping the dimension in which essential oils action, may be the link between the scientific domain and the esoteric realm of reality.

Essential oils are the most volatile molecules carrying the fragrances that entrance our olfactory sense and with it our whole sense of perception. There lays the soul of the plant.

These molecules are so unstable that they transform, disperse and eventually evaporate, they change their state so rapidly, so powerfully influenced by exterior conditions. And still, in this brief period of time when the essential oil is activated, its influence on our state of being is a complex phenomenon, simultaneously interfering with our organism on physical, psychological and emotional planes.

It's one mysterious substance, very hard to catch, but as such it's been the Holy Grail of perfumers and alchemists alike.

It is this transformative, dispersing nature that made this substance so mysterious and it is its infinitesimal quantity per plant that made it such a precious yield. It is no wonder that extracting these essential oils has been through millennia a practice so similar to that pursued by the alchemists in their search of extracting gold from inferior metals.

But from a therapeutic point of view, essential oils are just another type of plant extract, with nothing superior to alcohol macerates or brute water infusions. Each of them is employed in order to extract certain therapeutic compounds from the plant, the water soluble ones are captured in infusions, the light volatile ones are (most frequently) distilled into essential oils, while the heavy molecules are dissolvable in alcohol and other fixed oils. None of them contains the whole beneficial content of the plant, but each is the vessel of concentrated properties meant respond to particular issues.

Ancient knowledge of essential oils

The oldest written studies on plants and implicitly on their contained essential oils date as far back as 2-3000 BCE. Apparently, all ancient cultures had knowledge and veneration for the healing properties of wild herbs. The Indian Vedas list over 700 substances, among which we can find myrrh, coriander, ginger, cinnamon, plants that have been used therapeutically and ritualistically. This vast education was comprised in what became the basis of Ayurvedic medicine, one of the first holistic healing systems that was in accord with a holistic philosophy about life and all its integral parts, be it humans, plants or chemical elements.

The Chinese have also developed a vast encyclopedia of plants and their properties, including them in their rituals and extracting them into medicine. It was about the same animistic, cosmically interdependent perspective on life that sparked their interest into translating the correlations. They called in their knowledge of the energy points displayed all over the body, the yin-yang flux of the life force and their divination practice of I-Ching to succeed in creating a perfect and complete remedy. Learning and creating alongside nature, inspired them to advance the practice of acupuncture. Opium and ginger were the aromatic extracts mostly utilized by Asian cultures.

But among all, the Egyptians are the most famous for their balms and ointments, for an outstanding passion for fragrances as the ultimate instruments capable of preserving the human body, during and after life.

The concept of beauty was outstripped only by the divine and the divine nature was to be found in the essential purity. They had reached such perfection in their technique of extracting essential oils that the fragrances of frankincense and strap are still to be sensed in the tombs of pharaohs.

Their fame went so far that to this day, it is believed that the oldest documented extraction technique, of distilling the plant material, was developed and engraved in stones along the Nile valley. More recent, but less popularized discoveries have found older proofs of similar equipment designed and used about a thousand of years earlier by the Indians. Nevertheless, their legacy has been the primary lesson in perfumery, one that is still taught today.

Even the Bible mentions in several passages special recipes of anointing oils including essential extracts like cinnamon, myrrh, calamus, cassia and frankincense.

The ancients have created miraculous recipes, principles of combining plants that are implemented in today's pharmaceutical products. And among such treasures of the past lie multifunctional mixes of oils to be used therapeutically, as perfumes as well as internal medicine, oils that are best assimilated by our bodies. One such formula was implemented in the Egyptian kyphi, a blend of sixteen different plant extracts, balsamic and antiseptic, soothing for the nerves and nurturing for the soul, as well as an antidote to poison. It not only emulated their understanding of earthly life phenomenology but more than that, it reflected their insight into the esoteric sciences. The study of plants could not be discussed in the absence of astronomy, numerology and other sciences of divination, all of which were coordinates that guided the wise man in the creation of the healing potion.

The Greeks cultivated their own study of herbal remedies, but started by learning the basics already laid down before them by the Egyptians. Most of the resources that constitute the foundation of our current knowledge were documented by Greeks. They also created their own kyphi, called megaleion, that contained cinnamon, myrrh and cassia, to heal wounds and inflammations but also to envelope oneself in perfume.

From the Arabs, our universal culture has inherited a vast education on plants and especially on extracting their healing compounds. This is most likely by virtue of their passion for the rose. And with this came the desire to catch the essence of the miraculous plant, employing the technique of distillation and affixing the additional stage of cold processing for obtaining the purest extract.

This art of the Islam spread fast among Europeans that were fascinated by the exotic fragrances and were themselves inspired to use herbs native to their lands, like thyme, rosemary, sage, in the preparation of kindred essential oils.

How are essential oils absorbed by our bodies?

Though not dissolvable in water, the volatile oils are easily absorbed through the skin, through the blood vessels, entering the circuit and being transported to the organs, interacting with particular functions throughout the way.

That's why when you're having a dysfunction of a certain organ it is recommended to gently massage the skin area with the specific essential oil. For example, a disturbance of the liver can produce a general loss of balance and thus all sorts of disorders throughout the body. This machinery that processes every substance passing through our organism, that balances all internal processes, is also what the Chinese call the "eye opener", the essential tool controlling intuition and vision, the equilibrium of both mental and emotional states.

The spring ritual of detoxification is a cleansing procedure that happens inherently in your entire body and is aided by fresh detoxifying herbs like nettles. There are also essential oils to use with the same purpose – sage, cypress, lemon, chamomile, rose – they become effective when you rub your abdomen, penetrating through the surface skin cells, some are dispersed along the way, but most get to pass through the liver membrane, impressing the chemistry and functioning of the organ.

Blood vessels are responsible with transporting the essential oil molecules and dispersing them in your entire system. Being absorbed by your organism, they can be sensed emanating through the skin all over your body, surrounding it in their fragrance.

If you rub your heel with a garlic clove, after a while you'll feel the aroma in your mouth.

There are three ways in which the volatile oils permeate and get assimilated by your body, influencing its state – entering your blood they inter-relate directly with your chemistry, transforming it accordingly; they induct a certain mode of functioning depending on their particular properties, be it alert or sedated; and last but not least, when inhaled and catapulted into your brain, the essential plant compounds prompt a subtle and complex psychological shift, changing the active patterns. It is thus a concerted action, through various means – this is evidence of the intelligent and non-intrusive manner in which the natural medicine is designed to be harmoniously received by living organisms and participate in their healing. Moreover, when complementing the essential oils with other extracts of the same plant (water infusions, alcohol macerates), a whole congregated effect takes place inside your body, as all therapeutic properties are activated and when working in their original scheme the result is optimal.

The influence of essential oils on our state of being

The olfactory sense activates the same part of the brain that coordinates the functions of memory and emotion, the limbic system. It is smell that triggers memories – a unique combination and concentration of chemical elements, constrained by the particular conditions of that moment, that minute of that day that if by chance is met again; it would be able to reload in your consciousness, the entire universe of that moment.

Smelling helps us establish the locus, the time and space, provides the means of orientation on the scale of life events in a similar way in which it's employed by wild animals as a proficient scanner of their surroundings till kilometers away, as an instrument to establish their locus.

The olfactory channels are the direct routes in which you can administer a substance as to instantly affect your brain functions. The minuscule molecules of volatile oils are easily drawn inside your nostrils when breathing in, from there some are transmitted straight to the brain, while others are absorbed along the way.

Essential oils have been considered medicine for the mind since the beginnings of their use and study. Lavender oil has been reckoned to ease anxiety, while wild thyme was praised as the weed of the soul – the plant that cleared the mind and filled the heart with courage. Ancient Greeks were wearing it on their shields when marching to battles as well as burning it when practicing a ritual. Burning the plant breaks up its cells and frees the volatile compounds into the air – this is probably the oldest and simplest method to extract and use the essential oils.

Each compound of the plant's volatile oil confers a very subtle note to the overall effect on the mind of the breather. Each molecule is thus responsible for a smooth shift in the state of mind and the variety of these chemical elements corresponds to a mirroring diversity of effects. The primary alleviations that therapists have been searching for are stimuli for alertness and relaxation, but this binary couple is just the mainframe for a vast collection of intermediary tones. Some essential oils are prone to spark creativity, others induce feelings of nostalgia, some are sexual arousers, while others are depressants of desire – their area of action is such complex that our mind is not yet ready to grasp it. As it opens the dimension of the unseen, it brings forth a new understanding of the plane of reality.

As I've been writing, the action of essential oils is truly complex and sometimes their strategy is paradoxical. Some oils seem to have a tonic effect on some functions of our body and at the same time depressing on others, balancing our overall state almost magically, recreating a harmonious flow between the psychological and emotional planes. Essential oils that act in this modality are lemon balm or bergamot, that are relaxing the nervous system while uplifting your stamina; and in an opposite mirroring way, jasmine or neroli are uplifting the nerves activity and emotionally sedative.

As a general overview on the effects of essential oils on the state of mind, classifying simply according to this antipode – sedative / stimulant – a short list would look like this: Sedative compounds that are capable of alleviating stress, anxiety, insomnia: marjoram, lemon balm, sandalwood, bergamot, chamomile, valerian, hops / Stimulants, to boost up your energy level, to concentrate the nervously wrecked mind: rosemary, peppermint, basil, jasmine, ylang-ylang, clove, angelica.

Though of course this scheme is just a primary guideline, the subtle notes of one's psychology and in reverse of a plants specific chemical structure are of such versatility that cannot be contained in these two departments alone. This is just a mainframe for the physiological effect of the interaction with the volatile molecules floating in the air.

The psychological effect of a certain fragrance cannot be otherwise but personal and unique for each human being, depending on its chemical compatibility but as much, on one's previous experience with that particular smell namely on one's own associations. Studies into the relation between psychological states and specific smells, considered in this case triggers or promoters of moods, have revealed two different types of responses to odors. The basic reaction of our brain is instinctual – we are born with this pattern, it helps us distinguish nourishing from poisonous, friendly from dangerous. But we also use another method of scanning, one that we acquired through living and experiencing certain smells in certain moments – we ourselves along with our destiny, have put together involuntarily this pattern and we react precisely to the stimuli, some provoke nostalgia, others laughter, some make us angry or sad – each smell evokes a memory.

To truly understand the influence of essential oils on the body and mind you'd have to adopt a holistic approach, to search for impressions on the physical body but also on the psychological and emotional plane. And for this, healers have developed the science of aromatherapy. But this spectrum of knowledge has been disregarded and denigrated by conventional medicine, as were all alternative practices. The main contradiction derives from the premises that each use to structure their thesis – it is the holistic principle that is so hard to embrace by the institutionalized school of medicine, the fact that an emotional problem is implicitly reflected in a physical as well as mental condition.

Aromatherapy states that we can heal our body indirectly by working on our mind and heart – in parallel, acknowledged doctors would recommend for the same illness a direct intervention through pharmaceutically processed medicine or even surgery. This is obviously the imprint of the endless discussion on whether to approach therapy intrusively or non-intrusively, which after all derives from two different perspectives and thus conceptions about life itself. Are we to act brutally and interfere where we find something that doesn't fit our scheme or are we supposed to operate with more care and understanding so as not to disturb this complicated entanglement that defines our being in our attempt to heal it?

The beneficial properties of essential oils
Anti-inflammatory and antibacterial recipes

Our immune system benefits from any plant essential oil, one of the main processes that are encouraged by these volatile molecules is the production of white blood cells that refresh the whole system and help coping with infections. This antibacterial, antiseptic property that is a requisite of virtually all volatile oils is what brought forth this type of plant extract as an important medicinal value. During humanities troubled times, when large communities were struck by viral diseases as cholera and malaria, in periods of war or whenever there was a scarcity of clean water, essential oils have been intensively utilized as means of purifying and for stopping the spreading of epidemics. There's also the saying that whoever uses essential oils has a much stronger immune system and thus is less prone to infectious illnesses. Most proficient agents for combatting bacteria and viruses, in terms of concentration of effective chemical compounds, are the tea tree, eucalyptus, bergamot, basil, lavender, and rosemary and clove essential oils.

For skin inflammations, either bruises or eczema chamomile essential oil calms the area, soothes the skin, and relaxes the tissue. Lavender and yarrow are also beneficial, aiding an antibacterial, antiseptic effect.

Rubefacients that are able to unwind the muscles, warm up the area, dilate the blood vessels and increase the blood flow, thus releasing the inflammation. Essential oils like marjoram, camphor, juniper, pepper, rosemary is used in this type of conditions, soothing the swollen irritated tissue and loosening the stiffness.

When the inflammation occurs along the respiratory system, essential oils are the most effective medicine as they are best absorbed through inhalations, clearing the tract and making their way through the bronchi to the lungs, where they get exhaled. The bronchi are prompted to an increased secretion which itself assist the healing process. Eucalyptus, pine, thyme, myrrh, mint essential oils have an impressing instant effect, easing your breathing. Chamomile, bergamot, hyssop, cypress oils calm the spasms and the irritating sensations. While sage, tea tree and borneol oils act as antiseptics, natural antibiotics, eliminating the viral infection from the organism.

One of the main interactions of the essential oils with our body happens on a hormonal level; at the instant the volatile molecules penetrate into the blood system where they meet the hormones and enzymes. They act as regulators, reinstalling the hormonal balance, one of the main coordinates of a healthy body. There are some plants that are most beneficial for the reproductive system – rose and jasmine have a special relation to the genital organs, while hops and sage contain a plant hormone so similar in structure to our hormones that they literally pair perfectly when they meet. In addition, marjoram, basil, chamomile, lavender and jasmine calm the menstrual cramps. Bergamot, myrrh, tea tree and rose can be used with an anti-septic, anti-bacterial to eliminate infections.

Our bodies also give away unique fragranced imprints that reveal our chemistry, our momentary state of being along with the personal perfume note. This is the natural equation that guides the animals during the mating season.

But it does not reduce to sexual compatibility only – this scent, that has a specific recipe for each of us, defines our nature in chemical-biological terms, the way DNA scripts our genetics; thus, we can extend the analysis of compatibility by matching odors from the quest of finding a sexual partner to explaining almost all of life features. It is not as if the smell is the mainframe for understanding our biology, but our biology is imprinted in our smell and our sense of smell.

On the other hand, the effect of essential oils on a sexual plane has been for long studied, experimented and applied. It is and it has been the main purpose behind the development of the perfume industry, the main reason why we puff the chosen fragrance into the air and step inside its cloud before stepping out of the house, to be and to feel attractive. As such, there are essential oils that incite sexual arousal, aphrodisiacs like sage, neroli, black pepper, rose, jasmine, ylang-ylang, patchouli, cardamom, and sandalwood; as well as for decreasing desire, oils from herbs like marjoram and camphor.

Plant biology

Essential oils are to be found in all parts of a plant – citrus essential oil is extracted from the peel, in the case of rosemary it's contained in its leaves, for coriander oil we use the seeds, while for cinnamon we process the tree bark, the jasmine essential oil comes from the flowers and angelica oil is produced from the roots and seeds of the plant. But there is also the instance when different parts of the same plant are processed to obtain different essential oils compositions – the bitter orange tree is one such tributary as its leaves and twigs give away the petit grain, its fruit peels the original essential oil and its flowers contain the neroli oil.

All of these volatile compounds have a healing, soothing effect on the brain, on the heart and this way throughout the body – they're antidepressant, anti-inflammatory, and antispasmodic. And the neroli oil, so praised in ancient Egypt, has such a compatibility with our brain that it triggers it into producing more serotonin. (For the Neroli oil as well as in the case of rose essential oil, a huge quantity of plant matter is needed – the ratio is 1/1000).

The essential oil contained in one plant is rarely higher than 1% but it varies a lot from one type of plant to another and also in plants from the same family, to such an extent that in nutmeg, the concentration may be up to 10%.

Essential oils are soluble in alcohol and non-polar solutions, in oils, crèmes and waxes. They hardly dissolve in water and are of lower density. Most of them are colorless.

These minuscule molecules are contained in the plant's glands and they seem to direct the hormonal flow. They have the purpose of attracting or repelling insects, thus of promoting the functions of reproduction or protection. They start emanating their fragrance when the plant has reached maturity, at the time of spreading its pollen. Between the plant and the particular insect that pollinates it, there is bond that's been perfected in a long line of generations, the flower mimicking the most appealing odor for its matching insect, flirting with it. Thus, the symphony of fragrances is tributary and interdependent to the variety of insects. Some flowers open their treasure chests under the rays of the sun calling for the colorful butterflies and beetles, others in the shadow of night waiting for moths and other creatures of the dark.

And there are some flowers that have such a repelling stink for most of the living beings and yet so full of promises for some of the scavengers out there – these are the Carrion flowers or corpse flowers. As their name states it so clearly, they smell like cadavers, rotting flesh. They are so precise in their strategy that they developed their interior petals so as to resemble the texture of flesh and they also manipulate their temperature, raising it with the same purpose. And if this wasn't enough, certain species of corpse flowers even trap the fly or beetle inside to be sure that it's been covered in its pollen. Therefore, we have to be grateful to the tasteful insects out there, promoting the wonderful fragrances that mesmerize us.

And of course, there are other instances when the insects are repelled by certain smells that appear as beautiful perfumes to our noses. This is the case of the mint volatile oil, emanated by the leaves of the plant in order to fend off anyone who would dare to bite them. Same phenomenon can explain the odors of onion or garlic – it's recommended to plant garlic in your orchard at the base of young trees, to protect them against animals that would otherwise nibble the bark.

We also use plants following their principle, to get rid of any unwanted flying humming visitor. For this, the neem essential oil is effective for all species, but we also have discerned other particular incompatibilities that we exploit in our advantage – mosquitoes, flies or ticks are driven away by odors of essential compounds like mint, thyme, eucalyptus, rosemary, sage, geranium or lavender.

Essential oils compounds

Essential oils have mosaic structures, containing large numbers of individual compounds, some up to 60, while others are made up of over 100 different constituents. These chemical substances are recurring in various types of volatile oils, in distinct combinations, while some are unique and only to be found in a sole plant species. In pharmaceutical processing, one single compound is isolated in order to produce a specifically targeted medicine. But it has not been proved whether this selective manner is more efficient that the conjugated effect of all the constituting compounds.

Hydrocarbons are the most often met chemical elements in essential oils, constituted from molecules of carbon and hydrogen and classified in terpenes.

Examples: limonene, pinene, myrcene, azulene, thujane, cymene, cadinene, phellandrene.

Effects: antiviral, decongestant, antitumoral, antibacterial, stimulat, hepatoprotective.

Esters can be recognized by their sweet smell.

Examples: bornyl acetate, linalyl acetate, eugenol acetate, geraniol acetate.

Effects: anti-inflammatory, antispasmodic, antifungal, sedative.

Oxides exhibit the most stringent fragrances. One compound that is present in virtually any essential oil is an oxide, namely the 1,8-cineole.

Examples: linalool oxide, ascaridole, bisabolone oxide, sclareol oxide.

Effects: anti-inflammatory, general stimulant, expectorant.

Lactones are heavier compounds, more frequently found in plants that require cold pressing.

Examples: bergaptene, alantrolactone, psoralen, epinepetalactone, costuslactone, citroptene.

Effects: analgesic, hypotensive, sedative, antiviral, antimicrobial, antipyretic.

Alcohols are the most therapeutically valuable essential oils compounds.

Examples: borneol, menthol, linalol, citronellol, nerol, geraniol, santalol.

Effects: anti-inflammatory, antispasmodic, antiseptic, antimicrobial, tonifying.

When an essential oil is irritating for the skin but also for the mucous and the entire respiratory tract, that oil contains **phenols**. They have more or less the same range of action as alcohols but their effect is more profound.

Examples: eugenol, chavicol, thymol, carvacrol.

Effects: immune stimulating, antimicrobial, anaesthetic.

Aldehydes are also irritating but to a much lower degree than phenols. They present a sweet fruity fragrance and are extremely easily oxidated.

Examples: myrtenal, citronellal, citral, cuminaldehyde, benzaldehyde, cinnamaldehyde.

Effects: antimicrobial, antiviral, hypotensive, vasodilator, spasmolytic, sedative, calming, tonic.

Ketones are compounds that don't appear in the majority of essential oils. They differ a lot from the other families, especially because of their relatively stable structure and the fact that are almost insignificant in relation with the fragrance of the plant. Being a stable molecule, ketones cannot be easily assimilated by our liver; moreover a few types are also neurotoxic, like thujone.

Examples: menthone, fenchone,verbenon, carvone, thujone, camphor

Effects: antiviral, cell regenerating, neurotoxic, spasmolytic, mucolytic, analgesic.

Extraction

The methods used to extract essential oils are dependent on their specific chemical structure and that of the plant material. The water and water and steam distillation is the most practiced technique, as it is able to produce the optimal output. But still it is not recommended for fragile flower petals that require a more gracious apprehending – for them, the French promoted the method of enfleurage. A few types of volatile oils cannot be exposed to the amount of heat necessary for distillation without destroying their structure, thus another craft is engaged, that of cold pressing, conventionally called expression.

The technique of **enfleurage** was created and nurtured by the school of perfumery of Grasse, France. The flower petals are displayed on glass plates, previously prepared with a layer of odorless fat to absorb and preserve the volatile oils. But this is a time consuming practice as to concentrate a high number of essential oils, every 24 hours, the used flowers have to be carefully replaced with fresh ones, repeatedly for as long as the plants bloom during that season. It takes a lot of effort, patience and proficiency but the result of this method is praised by perfumers worldwide.

Expression is the simplest extraction option implemented exclusively for citrus oils. The essential oils contained in the peel are freed by perforating the glands. This is done by pressing the peel against a surface appointed with some sharp projections and squeezing a mixture of water and oil. The essential oil is separated through centrifugation.

Water distillation implies submerging the herbs in water and boiling the content, during this process the volatile compounds are freed and transformed into vapors that go through a cooling chamber and after that fall into a separator that directs the water residue into a vessel and the precious essential oil into its own. To perfect this method, steams were added to the equation – raising the plant material above the boiling water and exposing it to steam only. By this improvement, duration is shortened and the result is a higher concentration of oil, as the direct contact of boiling water is inevitably causing a considerable amount of volatile content to be damaged and lost. Heat is necessary to free the oils but in the same time it can also elicit their decomposition.

There is also a way to **macerate** the plants in a fixed cold pressed oil of choice – the extract will contain most of the plant properties. Though this is not a method to extract essential oils, the final mix will retain a considerable amount of the plant's original fragrance. Following the same rule as enfleurage, the fixed oil is subjected to several batches of fresh plants until sufficient impregnation.

A bottle of divine potion on the supermarket shelf

Until very recently essential oils have been the luxury of some and available for the many only in their purest form, that of a living fragranced field of flowers. And still this first hand use, a brief exposure to a fully blossomed field or an orchard, can have more of a healing effect than a precisely designed essential potion. One of the keys of developing an efficient medicine as well as a perfect perfume is to establish a harmonious mix of elements and to find that unique balance between the quantities of each plant.

A field of wild plants has the wisdom of nature imprinted in its recipe, it's been prepared in the perfect way, and it contains the most diverse bouquet, with all stringent aromas and subtle notes equilibrated. To reenact such complex and fragile unity of chemical compounds, the man cannot rely solely on its scientific, rational mind processes, but such performance requires the hand of an artist. To extract essential oils is a craft, but to mix them into recreating the moment of early morning in the mountains when the sharp cold air brings along the fresh pine fragrance and the sweet lavender perfume, when the atmosphere is wet and you can smell the resin on the trees, the soil, the wet leaves on the forest ground – this is art. It is not only a scent you are reproducing; it is a whole state of being – your nose senses the difference, your brain knows it.

And to return to the common man one hundred years ago – for him essential oils are not just something that he hasn't used, hasn't seen, hasn't smelled, but they are something that most probably he hasn't heard of, but as myth, a story of no real experienced proof. These were not simples that every grandma used to prepare from the plants that herself collected. Because even the simplest methods of extracting volatile oils are pursued using a minimum of technical equipment and a huge amount of base plant matter, not to mention the effort and time.

Therefore, the precious oils were too expansive for anyone but the nobles and royals. For many millennia they were produced to support the privilege and trifles of the wealthy class as well as to preserve an ancient knowledge. This medicinal practice was used to cure illnesses but most importantly, essential oils have been involved in religious rituals, all over the earth, ever since man discovered this miraculous liquid, in the times of the many gods. All ancient cultures made use of herbal scents to accompany their rituals, to create a bridge between the material reality and the ethereal world dimension of life. What other vehicle than the volatile molecule of the sacred plants could succeed better in connecting the soul of the mortals to that of the divine?

It must be a divine molecule itself - for that I was calling it earlier the soul of the plant. By inhaling it, we are under its effect – it transposes us into a fertile state of mind for us to be able to perceive sanctity, the surreal dimension of reality, the realm of saints and gods.

Just try to imagine this context for a moment – the times when a small bottle of essential rose oil was among the very few you could find around the whole world and it was worth a fortune to use just one drop of it. And then open your internet search browser and check out the multitude of shops selling at this very moment essential oils to be bought with one click and shipped for thousands of kilometers across the globe. There is a troubling discrepancy between what our ancestors were pricing almost as invaluable and the way we are appreciating this healing gift of plants now.

Of course, if we choose to look this way, we must acknowledge the human evolution and the balancing, leveling of the social strata along with the leaps of constant technological improvements. This made it easier to process large quantities of plant matter and reduced the costs enough to make it a profitable industry for all to benefit from it. The business is sustained by the high demand from the food industry, pharmacology and cosmetics. But this makes it profitable enough as to sustain the production of essential oils extracted from plants that are not that solicited on the market, action that is unprofitable in itself. And it is amazing that beneficial that such a variety of products from so far away corners of the planet are accessible for us, if we use them wisely.

Firstly, the plants that will be most helpful are the ones to be found in your close surroundings, the same environment your body's grown accustomed to. Those plants shared the same air, the same water, complementary to everything else you consume, thus are most compatible with your needs.

You may find an exotic equivalent from another continent that may contain a much higher concentration of the compound you're searching for but still, your native plant will exhibit the unique chemical structure to supply your receptors with their adequate input.

The price of one bottle of essential oil seems low now but in fact is sky high when you consider the number of plants that is used to produce it. It's true that rose oil is one of the most difficult to obtain, as its concentration per flower is so small – it takes about 100 kg of petals for only about 30 g of volatile substance. Other plants give a higher oil yield but still, the quantity of plants consumed in this process is overwhelming.

Thus, you should value your essential oil drop accordingly. One spilled drop would be the equivalent of a whole day of collecting flowers. It's hard to praise a product with a cheap market value, same way as it is incomprehensible for a civilized city citizen to regard water as an invaluable resource, unless he travels to the African desert for example to experience water scarcity on his own body. So, to estimate the value of just one plant you have look more profoundly, skip the marketing and price tag, envision the natural resources and the complex phenomenon that took place in order for you to enjoy the precious healing gift.

Nowadays everything we use is perfumed, from the clothes we wear to the toilet paper we use, every object, every indoor, we use it to disperse nasty odors, to compensate the tobacco smell, to make us more attractive, to feel clean, we spray, we puff, we burn fragranced candles and sticks. More than we use it, we abuse it. We almost feel unsafe when there's no perfume in the air. And most of the aromas that are dispersed in the air today are artificial. We don't realize but by doing so, we abuse our noses and our olfactory sense is one of the most precious, as among all our senses this is the one that intermediates our contact with the immediate reality.

We might think that vision is the primary guiding instrument but our animal organism is better constructed to rely on smell as the main orienting sense. It's an inheritance from the times we were climbing trees and eating bananas and its function hasn't changed much during our luminous evolution. Bombarding our noses with all sorts of perfumes, ignoring the way one fragrance mixes with the others, never minding that each compound has a subtle but strong effect on our mind and body, guides us only to a disoriented, distressed state of being.

Cherish and be aware of your sense of smell.
Praise the plants as they sustain your life.
Let the essential oils guide you.